My 12 Week
HEALTH
JOURNAL

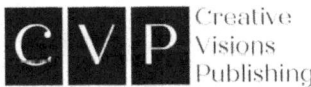
Creative Visions Publishing

ISBN: 978-1-312-72904-9

This Journal Belongs To:

Contact Details:

📞 ....

✉️ ....

📮 ....

We love hearing from you!

Please take a moment to leave us a review. Let us know how this book is serving you and what we can do to serve you better through future editions.

An email from you would be greatly appreciated!
Title it "My 12 Week Health Planner" and we will send you a free gift!

✉ creativevisionspublishing@gmail.com

⬜ @creativevisionspublishing

Ⓕ @creativevisionspublishing

We wish you many years of perfect health!

Enjoy logging!

My Weight Goals

Date: ....

CURRENT:

GOALS:

WEIGHT:

WEIGHT:

YOU'VE TOTALLY GOT THIS!

Thoughts & Plans About The Next 12 Weeks

....
....
....
....
....
....
....
....
....
....
....
....
....
....
....
....
....
....
....
....
....
....
....
....
....
....
....
....
....
....
....
....

Daily Health Log

Date: ....

FOOD LOG

Breakfast:

Lunch:

Dinner:

Snacks:

YES   NO

SUGAR   YES   NO

EXERCISE   YES   NO

HYDRATION

0.5L   1.0L   1.5L   2.0L

Length of Sleep (Hours):   ① ② ③ ④ ⑤ ⑥ ⑦ ⑧ ⑨ ⑩

Win of the Day: ....
....

Goals for Tomorrow: ....
....

Notes: ....
....

Today's Mood: 😠 😢 🙁 😐 🙂 😀 😄   Day's Rating: ☆☆☆☆☆☆

Daily Health Log

Date: ....

FOOD LOG

Breakfast:

Lunch:

Dinner:

Snacks:

YES   NO

SUGAR   YES   NO

EXERCISE   YES   NO

HYDRATION

0.5L   1.0L   1.5L   2.0L

Length of Sleep (Hours): (1) (2) (3) (4) (5) (6) (7) (8) (9) (10)

Win of the Day: ....
....

Goals for Tomorrow: ....
....

Notes: ....
....
....

Today's Mood: 😠 😟 😐 😑 🙂 😄 😂   Day's Rating: ☆☆☆☆☆☆

Date: ....

FOOD LOG

Breakfast:

YES NO

SUGAR YES NO

EXERCISE YES NO

Lunch:

Dinner:

HYDRATION

Snacks:

0.5L 1.0L 1.5L 2.0L

Length of Sleep (Hours): (1) (2) (3) (4) (5) (6) (7) (8) (9) (10)

Win of the Day: ....

Goals for Tomorrow: ....

Notes: ....

Today's Mood: 😠 😞 🙁 😐 🙂 😄 😁   Day's Rating: ☆☆☆☆☆

Date: ....

FOOD LOG

Breakfast:

YES   NO

SUGAR YES   NO

EXERCISE YES   NO

Lunch:

HYDRATION

Dinner:

Snacks:

0.5L   1.0L   1.5L   2.0L

Length of Sleep (Hours): ① ② ③ ④ ⑤ ⑥ ⑦ ⑧ ⑨ ⑩

Win of the Day: ....
....

Goals for Tomorrow: ....
....
....

Notes: ....
....
....

Today's Mood: 😠 😞 🙁 😐 🙂 😀 😄   Day's Rating: ☆☆☆☆☆☆

Daily Health Log

Date: ....

FOOD LOG

Breakfast:

YES   NO

SUGAR   YES   NO

EXERCISE   YES   NO

Lunch:

Dinner:

HYDRATION

0.5L   1.0L   1.5L   2.0L

Snacks:

Length of Sleep (Hours): (1) (2) (3) (4) (5) (6) (7) (8) (9) (10)

Win of the Day: ....

....

Goals for Tomorrow: ....

....

Notes: ....

....

....

Today's Mood: 😠 😟 🙁 😐 🙂 😃 😄   Day's Rating: ☆☆☆☆☆

Date: ....

FOOD LOG

Breakfast:

Lunch:

Dinner:

Snacks:

YES   NO

SUGAR   YES   NO

EXERCISE   YES   NO

HYDRATION

0.5L   1.0L   1.5L   2.0L

Length of Sleep (Hours): ① ② ③ ④ ⑤ ⑥ ⑦ ⑧ ⑨ ⑩

Win of the Day: ....

Goals for Tomorrow: ....

Notes: ....

Today's Mood: 😠 😢 😕 😐 🙂 😃 😂   Day's Rating: ☆☆☆☆☆☆

FOOD LOG

Date: ....

Breakfast:

YES   NO

SUGAR   YES   NO

EXERCISE   YES   NO

Lunch:

Dinner:

HYDRATION

Snacks:

0.5L   1.0L   1.5L   2.0L

Length of Sleep (Hours): ① ② ③ ④ ⑤ ⑥ ⑦ ⑧ ⑨ ⑩

Win of the Day: ....
....

Goals for Tomorrow: ....
....

Notes: ....
....
....

Today's Mood: 😠 😟 🙁 😐 🙂 😄 😁   Day's Rating: ☆ ☆ ☆ ☆ ☆

Weekly Weigh-In

Wk 1

Date: ....

WEIGHT:

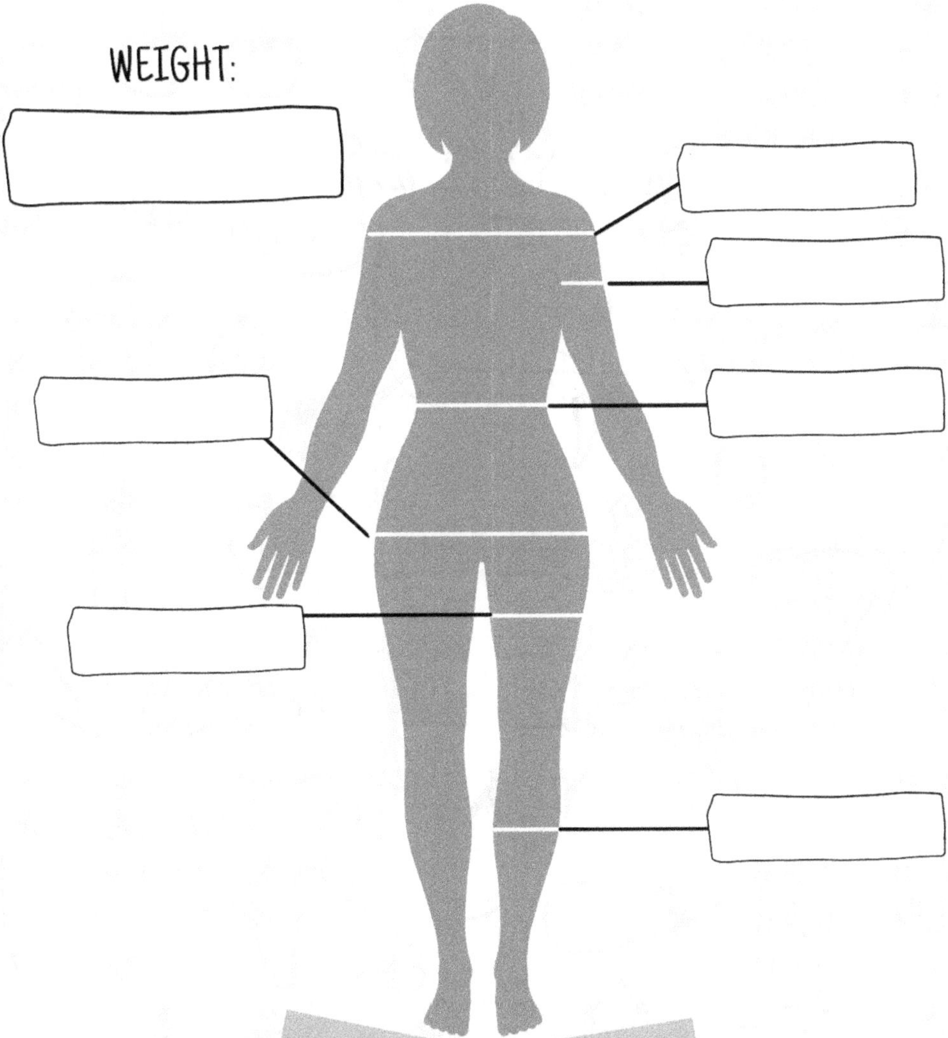

"It does not matter how slowly you go, as long as you don't stop!"

Daily Health Log

Wk 2

Date: ....

FOOD LOG

Breakfast:

Lunch:

Dinner:

Snacks:

YES   NO

SUGAR   YES   NO

EXERCISE   YES   NO

HYDRATION

0.5L   1.0L   1.5L   2.0L

Length of Sleep (Hours): (1) (2) (3) (4) (5) (6) (7) (8) (9) (10)

Win of the Day: ....
....

Goals for Tomorrow: ....
....

Notes: ....
....
....

Today's Mood: 😠😟☹️😐🙂😃😄   Day's Rating: ☆☆☆☆☆

Date: ....

FOOD LOG

Breakfast:

YES   NO

SUGAR   YES   NO

EXERCISE   YES   NO

Lunch:

Dinner:

HYDRATION

Snacks:

0.5L   1.0L   1.5L   2.0L

Length of Sleep (Hours): (1) (2) (3) (4) (5) (6) (7) (8) (9) (10)

Win of the Day: ....
....

Goals for Tomorrow: ....
....

Notes: ....
....
....

Today's Mood: 😠 😢 😟 😐 🙂 😁 😂   Day's Rating: ☆☆☆☆☆

Date: ....

FOOD LOG

Breakfast:

Lunch:

Dinner:

Snacks:

YES NO

SUGAR YES NO

EXERCISE YES NO

HYDRATION

0.5L   1.0L   1.5L   2.0L

Length of Sleep (Hours): ① ② ③ ④ ⑤ ⑥ ⑦ ⑧ ⑨ ⑩

Win of the Day: ....

....

Goals for Tomorrow: ....

....

Notes: ....

....

....

Today's Mood: 😠 😞 😣 😐 🙂 😄 😁   Day's Rating: ☆☆☆☆☆☆

Date: ....

FOOD LOG

Breakfast:

Lunch:

Dinner:

Snacks:

YES   NO

SUGAR   YES   NO

EXERCISE   YES   NO

HYDRATION

0.5L   1.0L   1.5L   2.0L

Length of Sleep (Hours): ① ② ③ ④ ⑤ ⑥ ⑦ ⑧ ⑨ ⑩

Win of the Day: ....
....

Goals for Tomorrow: ....
....

Notes: ....
....
....

Today's Mood: 😠 😟 🙁 😐 🙂 😃 😂   Day's Rating: ☆☆☆☆☆

Date: ....

FOOD LOG

Breakfast:

YES NO

SUGAR   YES   NO

EXERCISE   YES   NO

Lunch:

HYDRATION

Dinner:

Snacks:

0.5L   1.0L   1.5L   2.0L

Length of Sleep (Hours): (1) (2) (3) (4) (5) (6) (7) (8) (9) (10)

Win of the Day: ....

....

Goals for Tomorrow: ....

....

Notes: ....

....

....

Today's Mood: 😠 😟 🙁 😐 🙂 😄 😁   Day's Rating: ☆☆☆☆☆

Date: ....

FOOD LOG

Breakfast:

Lunch:

Dinner:

Snacks:

YES   NO

SUGAR   YES   NO

EXERCISE   YES   NO

HYDRATION

0.5L   1.0L   1.5L   2.0L

Length of Sleep (Hours): 1 2 3 4 5 6 7 8 9 10

Win of the Day: ....
....

Goals for Tomorrow: ....
....

Notes: ....
....
....

Today's Mood: 😠 😢 😕 😐 🙂 😃 😂   Day's Rating: ☆☆☆☆☆☆

Date: ....

FOOD LOG

Breakfast:

YES   NO

Lunch:

SUGAR   YES   NO

EXERCISE   YES   NO

Dinner:

HYDRATION

Snacks:

0.5L   1.0L   1.5L   2.0L

Length of Sleep (Hours): ① ② ③ ④ ⑤ ⑥ ⑦ ⑧ ⑨ ⑩

Win of the Day: ....

Goals for Tomorrow: ....

Notes: ....

Today's Mood: 😠 😢 🙁 😐 🙂 😄 😁   Day's Rating: ☆ ☆ ☆ ☆ ☆

Date: ....

WEIGHT:

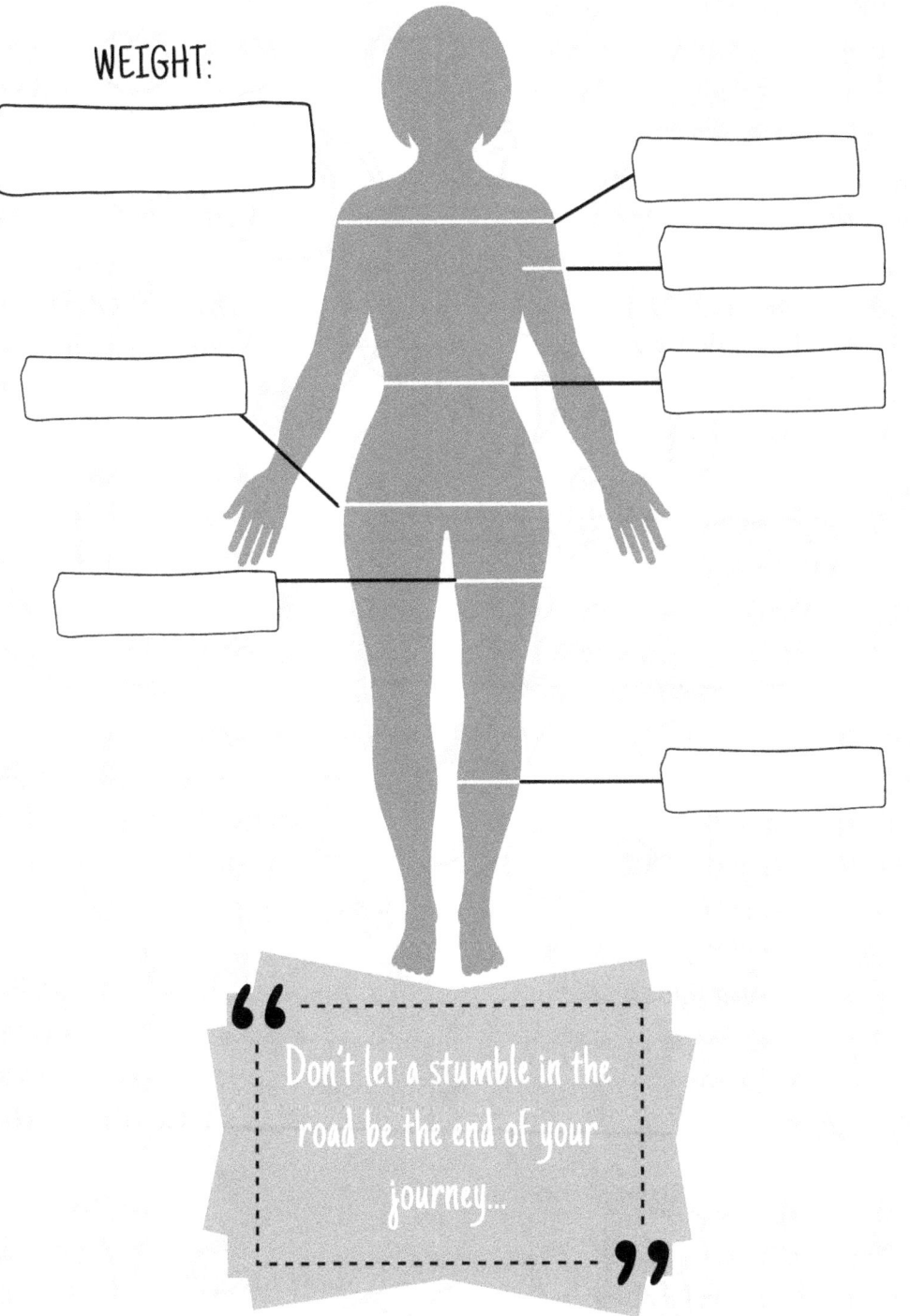

> Don't let a stumble in the road be the end of your journey...

Date: ....

FOOD LOG

Breakfast:

Lunch:

Dinner:

Snacks:

YES NO

SUGAR YES NO

EXERCISE YES NO

HYDRATION

0.5L 1.0L 1.5L 2.0L

Length of Sleep (Hours): (1) (2) (3) (4) (5) (6) (7) (8) (9) (10)

Win of the Day: ....

Goals for Tomorrow: ....

Notes: ....

Today's Mood: 😠 😦 😕 😐 🙂 😁 😄   Day's Rating: ☆☆☆☆☆☆

Date: ....

FOOD LOG

Breakfast:

YES   NO

SUGAR   YES   NO

EXERCISE   YES   NO

Lunch:

Dinner:

HYDRATION

Snacks:

0.5L   1.0L   1.5L   2.0L

Length of Sleep (Hours): ① ② ③ ④ ⑤ ⑥ ⑦ ⑧ ⑨ ⑩

Win of the Day: ....
....

Goals for Tomorrow: ....
....

Notes: ....
....
....

Today's Mood: 😠 😟 😕 😐 🙂 😄 😂   Day's Rating: ☆☆☆☆☆

Date: ....

FOOD LOG

Breakfast:

YES   NO

SUGAR   YES   NO

EXERCISE   YES   NO

Lunch:

Dinner:

HYDRATION

Snacks:

0.5L   1.0L   1.5L   2.0L

Length of Sleep (Hours):   ① ② ③ ④ ⑤ ⑥ ⑦ ⑧ ⑨ ⑩

Win of the Day: ....
....
....

Goals for Tomorrow: ....
....
....

Notes: ....
....
....
....

Today's Mood: 😠 😞 🙁 😐 🙂 😄 😁   Day's Rating: ☆☆☆☆☆

Date: ....

FOOD LOG

Breakfast:

Lunch:

Dinner:

Snacks:

YES NO

SUGAR YES NO

EXERCISE YES NO

HYDRATION

0.5L 1.0L 1.5L 2.0L

Length of Sleep (Hours): ① ② ③ ④ ⑤ ⑥ ⑦ ⑧ ⑨ ⑩

Win of the Day: ....
....

Goals for Tomorrow: ....
....

Notes: ....
....
....

Today's Mood: 😠 😟 😣 😐 🙂 😄 😆   Day's Rating: ☆☆☆☆☆☆

Date: ....

FOOD LOG

Breakfast:

YES NO

SUGAR YES NO

EXERCISE YES NO

Lunch:

Dinner:

HYDRATION

Snacks:

0.5L 1.0L 1.5L 2.0L

Length of Sleep (Hours): ① ② ③ ④ ⑤ ⑥ ⑦ ⑧ ⑨ ⑩

Win of the Day: ....
....

Goals for Tomorrow: ....
....
....

Notes: ....
....
....

Today's Mood: 😠 😞 🙁 😐 🙂 😀 😁   Day's Rating: ☆☆☆☆☆

Date: ....

FOOD LOG

Breakfast:

Lunch:

Dinner:

Snacks:

YES   NO

SUGAR   YES   NO

EXERCISE   YES   NO

HYDRATION

0.5L   1.0L   1.5L   2.0L

Length of Sleep (Hours): 1 2 3 4 5 6 7 8 9 10

Win of the Day: ....
....

Goals for Tomorrow: ....
....

Notes: ....
....
....

Today's Mood: 😠 😦 😕 😐 🙂 😄 😁   Day's Rating: ☆☆☆☆☆☆

Date: ....

FOOD LOG

Breakfast:

YES NO

SUGAR YES NO

EXERCISE YES NO

Lunch:

Dinner:

HYDRATION

Snacks:

0.5L 1.0L 1.5L 2.0L

Length of Sleep (Hours): ① ② ③ ④ ⑤ ⑥ ⑦ ⑧ ⑨ ⑩

Win of the Day: ....
....

Goals for Tomorrow: ....
....
....

Notes: ....
....
....

Today's Mood: 😠 😟 🙁 😐 🙂 😄 😆   **Day's Rating:** ☆ ☆ ☆ ☆ ☆

Date: ....

WEIGHT:

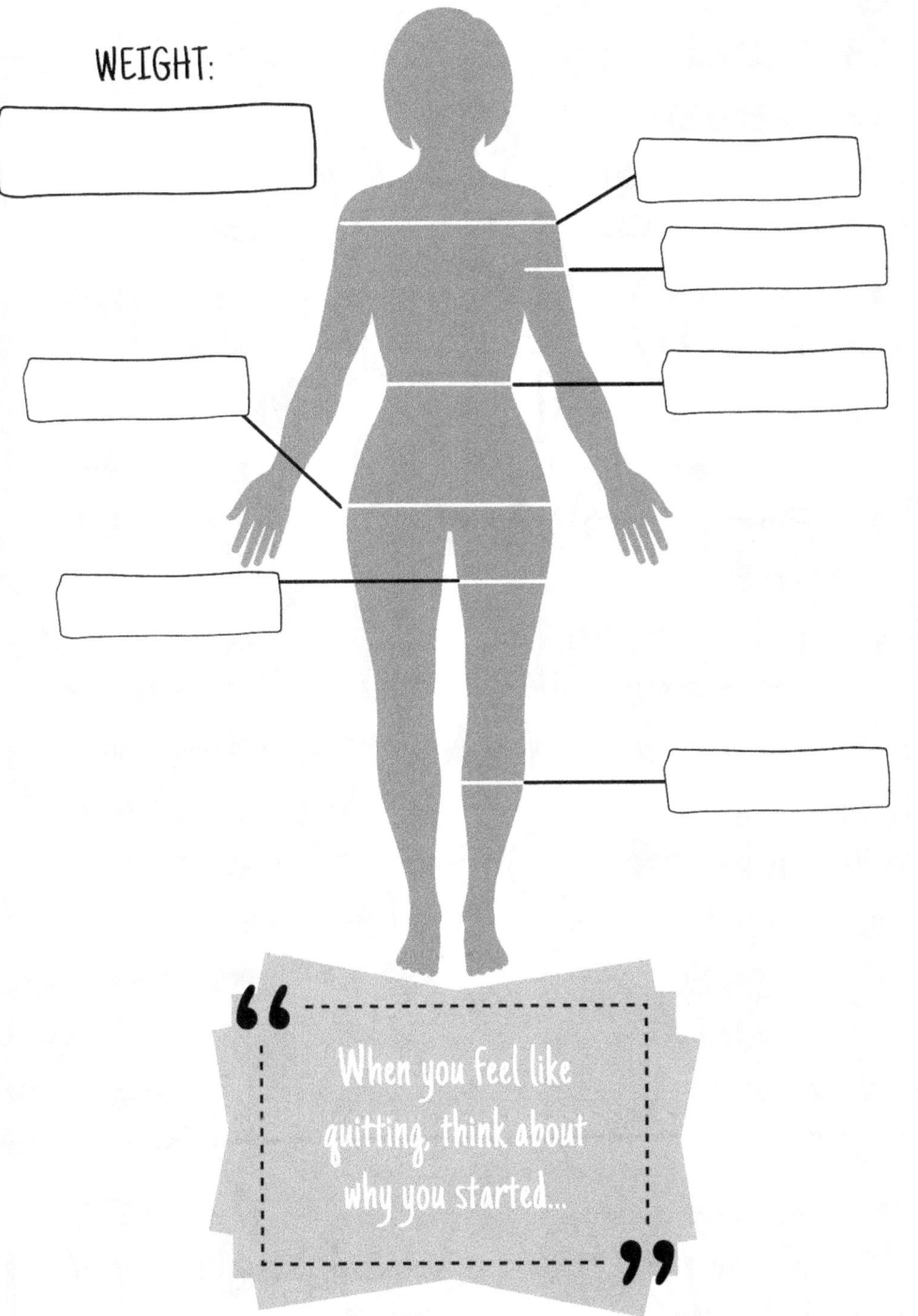

> When you feel like quitting, think about why you started...

Date: ....

FOOD LOG

Breakfast:

YES   NO

SUGAR   YES   NO

EXERCISE   YES   NO

Lunch:

Dinner:

HYDRATION

Snacks:

0.5L   1.0L   1.5L   2.0L

Length of Sleep (Hours): (1) (2) (3) (4) (5) (6) (7) (8) (9) (10)

Win of the Day: ....
....

Goals for Tomorrow: ....
....

Notes: ....
....
....

Today's Mood: 😠 😢 ☹️ 😐 🙂 😄 😆   Day's Rating: ☆☆☆☆☆

Daily Health Log

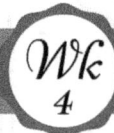

Date: ....

FOOD LOG

Breakfast:

YES   NO

SUGAR   YES   NO

EXERCISE   YES   NO

Lunch:

Dinner:

HYDRATION

Snacks:

0.5L   1.0L   1.5L   2.0L

Length of Sleep (Hours): (1)(2)(3)(4)(5)(6)(7)(8)(9)(10)

Win of the Day: ....
....

Goals for Tomorrow: ....
....

Notes: ....
....
....

Today's Mood: 😠 😢 😟 😐 🙂 😃 😂   Day's Rating: ☆☆☆☆☆☆

Date: ....

FOOD LOG

Breakfast:

YES   NO

Lunch:

SUGAR   YES   NO

EXERCISE   YES   NO

Dinner:

HYDRATION

Snacks:

0.5L   1.0L   1.5L   2.0L

Length of Sleep (Hours): ① ② ③ ④ ⑤ ⑥ ⑦ ⑧ ⑨ ⑩

Win of the Day: ....

....

Goals for Tomorrow: ....

....

Notes: ....

....

....

Today's Mood: 😠 😟 🙁 😐 🙂 😃 😄   Day's Rating: ☆☆☆☆☆

Date: ....

FOOD LOG

Breakfast:

 YES   NO

SUGAR   YES   NO

EXERCISE   YES   NO

Lunch:

Dinner:

HYDRATION

Snacks:

0.5L   1.0L   1.5L   2.0L

Length of Sleep (Hours): ① ② ③ ④ ⑤ ⑥ ⑦ ⑧ ⑨ ⑩

Win of the Day: ....
....

Goals for Tomorrow: ....
....

Notes: ....
....
....

Today's Mood: 😠 😣 ☹️ 😐 🙂 😀 😂   Day's Rating: ☆☆☆☆☆☆

Wk 4

Date: ....

FOOD LOG

Breakfast:

YES   NO

Lunch:

SUGAR   YES   NO

EXERCISE   YES   NO

Dinner:

HYDRATION

Snacks:

0.5L   1.0L   1.5L   2.0L

Length of Sleep (Hours): (1) (2) (3) (4) (5) (6) (7) (8) (9) (10)

Win of the Day: ....
....

Goals for Tomorrow: ....
....

Notes: ....
....
....

Today's Mood: 😠 😟 🙁 😐 🙂 😄 😁   Day's Rating: ☆☆☆☆☆

Date: ....

FOOD LOG

Breakfast:

YES   NO

SUGAR   YES   NO

EXERCISE   YES   NO

Lunch:

Dinner:

HYDRATION

Snacks:

0.5L   1.0L   1.5L   2.0L

Length of Sleep (Hours): ① ② ③ ④ ⑤ ⑥ ⑦ ⑧ ⑨ ⑩

Win of the Day: ....
....

Goals for Tomorrow: ....
....

Notes: ....
....
....

Today's Mood: 😠 😢 🙁 😐 🙂 😃 😆   Day's Rating: ☆☆☆☆☆☆

Date: ....

FOOD LOG

Breakfast:

Lunch:

Dinner:

Snacks:

YES NO

SUGAR YES NO

EXERCISE YES NO

HYDRATION

0.5L 1.0L 1.5L 2.0L

Length of Sleep (Hours): ① ② ③ ④ ⑤ ⑥ ⑦ ⑧ ⑨ ⑩

Win of the Day: ....

Goals for Tomorrow: ....

Notes: ....

Today's Mood: 😠 😟 🙁 😐 🙂 😃 😄   Day's Rating: ☆☆☆☆☆

Weekly Weigh-In

Wk 4

Date: ....

WEIGHT:

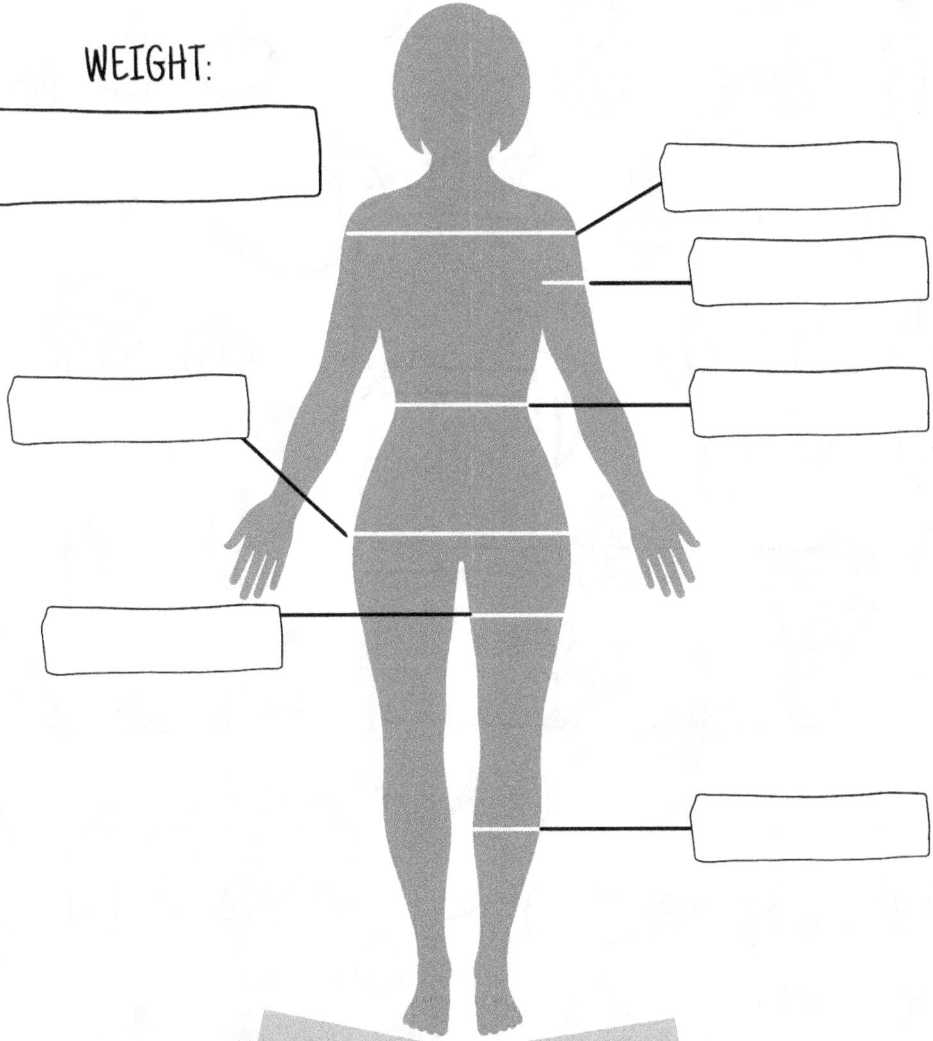

“ Fall seven times, stand up eight... ”

Date: ....

FOOD LOG

Breakfast:

Lunch:

Dinner:

Snacks:

YES   NO

SUGAR   YES   NO

EXERCISE   YES   NO

HYDRATION

0.5L   1.0L   1.5L   2.0L

Length of Sleep (Hours): ① ② ③ ④ ⑤ ⑥ ⑦ ⑧ ⑨ ⑩

Win of the Day: ....
....
....

Goals for Tomorrow: ....
....
....

Notes: ....
....
....

Today's Mood: 😠 😟 🙁 😐 🙂 😀 😆   Day's Rating: ☆☆☆☆☆☆

Date: ....

FOOD LOG

Breakfast:

Lunch:

Dinner:

Snacks:

YES   NO

SUGAR   YES   NO

EXERCISE   YES   NO

HYDRATION

0.5L   1.0L   1.5L   2.0L

Length of Sleep (Hours): ① ② ③ ④ ⑤ ⑥ ⑦ ⑧ ⑨ ⑩

Win of the Day: ....
....

Goals for Tomorrow: ....
....

Notes: ....
....
....

Today's Mood: 😠 😟 😕 😐 🙂 😃 😄   Day's Rating: ☆☆☆☆☆

Date: ....

FOOD LOG

Breakfast:

Lunch:

Dinner:

Snacks:

YES   NO

SUGAR   YES   NO

EXERCISE   YES   NO

HYDRATION

0.5L   1.0L   1.5L   2.0L

Length of Sleep (Hours): ① ② ③ ④ ⑤ ⑥ ⑦ ⑧ ⑨ ⑩

Win of the Day: ....

Goals for Tomorrow: ....

Notes: ....

Today's Mood: 😠 😞 😕 😐 🙂 😃 😄   Day's Rating: ☆☆☆☆☆

Date: ....

FOOD LOG

Breakfast:

YES   NO

Lunch:

SUGAR   YES   NO

EXERCISE   YES   NO

Dinner:

HYDRATION

Snacks:

0.5L   1.0L   1.5L   2.0L

Length of Sleep (Hours): ① ② ③ ④ ⑤ ⑥ ⑦ ⑧ ⑨ ⑩

Win of the Day: ....
....

Goals for Tomorrow: ....
....

Notes: ....
....
....

Today's Mood: 😠 😟 😕 😐 🙂 😃 😂   Day's Rating: ☆☆☆☆☆

Date:

FOOD LOG

Breakfast:

Lunch:

Dinner:

Snacks:

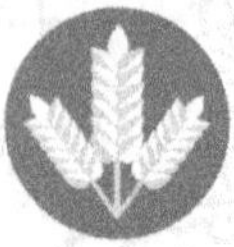

YES   NO

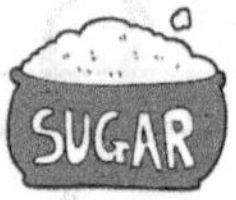

SUGAR   YES   NO

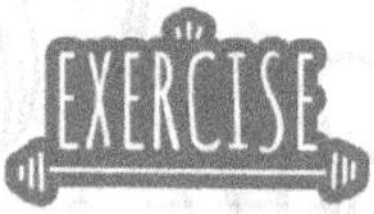

EXERCISE   YES   NO

HYDRATION

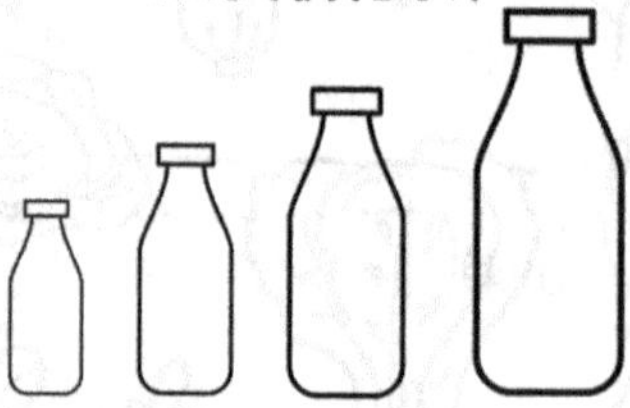

0.5L   1.0L   1.5L   2.0L

Length of Sleep (Hours): 1 2 3 4 5 6 7 8 9 10

Win of the Day:

Goals for Tomorrow:

Notes:

Today's Mood: Day's Rating: ☆☆☆☆☆

Daily Health Log

Wk 5

Date: ....

FOOD LOG

Breakfast:

Lunch:

Dinner:

Snacks:

YES NO

SUGAR YES NO

EXERCISE YES NO

HYDRATION

0.5L 1.0L 1.5L 2.0L

Length of Sleep (Hours): ① ② ③ ④ ⑤ ⑥ ⑦ ⑧ ⑨ ⑩

Win of the Day: ....
....

Goals for Tomorrow: ....
....

Notes: ....
....
....

Today's Mood: 😠 😟 😕 😐 🙂 😄 😂   Day's Rating: ☆☆☆☆☆☆

Daily Health Log

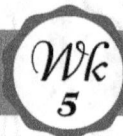

Wk 5

Date: ....

FOOD LOG

Breakfast:

Lunch:

Dinner:

Snacks:

YES NO

SUGAR YES NO

EXERCISE YES NO

HYDRATION

0.5L 1.0L 1.5L 2.0L

Length of Sleep (Hours): ① ② ③ ④ ⑤ ⑥ ⑦ ⑧ ⑨ ⑩

Win of the Day: ....
....

Goals for Tomorrow: ....
....

Notes: ....
....
....

Today's Mood: 😠 😞 🙁 😐 🙂 😄 😂   Day's Rating: ☆☆☆☆☆

Weekly Weigh-In

Wk
5

Date: ....

WEIGHT:

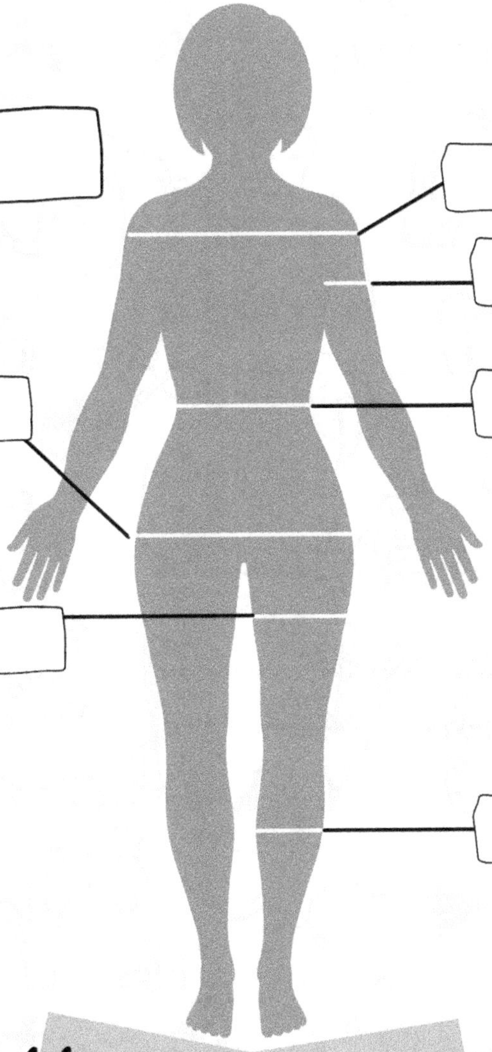

“ Every step is progress,
no matter how small... ”

Date: ....

FOOD LOG

Breakfast:

Lunch:

Dinner:

Snacks:

 YES NO

SUGAR YES NO

EXERCISE YES NO

HYDRATION

0.5L 1.0L 1.5L 2.0L

Length of Sleep (Hours): ① ② ③ ④ ⑤ ⑥ ⑦ ⑧ ⑨ ⑩

Win of the Day: ....

Goals for Tomorrow: ....

Notes: ....

Today's Mood: 😠 😟 🙁 😐 🙂 😄 😁   **Day's Rating:** ☆☆☆☆☆

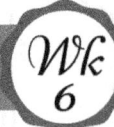
Date: ....

FOOD LOG

Breakfast:

Lunch:

Dinner:

Snacks:

YES   NO

SUGAR   YES   NO

EXERCISE   YES   NO

HYDRATION

0.5L   1.0L   1.5L   2.0L

Length of Sleep (Hours): ① ② ③ ④ ⑤ ⑥ ⑦ ⑧ ⑨ ⑩

Win of the Day: ....

Goals for Tomorrow: ....

Notes: ....

Today's Mood: 😠 🙁 😕 😐 🙂 😃 😄   Day's Rating: ☆☆☆☆☆☆

Date: ....

FOOD LOG

Breakfast:

Lunch:

Dinner:

Snacks:

YES   NO

SUGAR   YES   NO

EXERCISE   YES   NO

HYDRATION

0.5L   1.0L   1.5L   2.0L

Length of Sleep (Hours): ① ② ③ ④ ⑤ ⑥ ⑦ ⑧ ⑨ ⑩

Win of the Day: ....

Goals for Tomorrow: ....

Notes: ....

Today's Mood: 😠 😞 🙁 😐 🙂 😀 😄   Day's Rating: ☆☆☆☆☆

Date: ....

FOOD LOG

Breakfast:

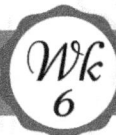 YES NO

SUGAR YES NO

EXERCISE YES NO

Lunch:

Dinner:

HYDRATION

Snacks:

0.5L 1.0L 1.5L 2.0L

Length of Sleep (Hours): ① ② ③ ④ ⑤ ⑥ ⑦ ⑧ ⑨ ⑩

Win of the Day: ....
....

Goals for Tomorrow: ....
....

Notes: ....
....
....

Today's Mood: 😠 😟 😕 😐 🙂 😃 😆   Day's Rating: ☆☆☆☆☆☆

Date: ....

FOOD LOG

Breakfast:

YES NO

Lunch:

SUGAR YES NO

EXERCISE YES NO

Dinner:

HYDRATION

Snacks:

0.5L 1.0L 1.5L 2.0L

Length of Sleep (Hours): ① ② ③ ④ ⑤ ⑥ ⑦ ⑧ ⑨ ⑩

Win of the Day: ....
....

Goals for Tomorrow: ....
....
....

Notes: ....
....
....

Today's Mood: 😠 😞 🙁 😐 🙂 😀 😄   **Day's Rating:** ☆☆☆☆☆

Date: ....

FOOD LOG

Breakfast:

Lunch:

Dinner:

Snacks:

YES   NO

SUGAR   YES   NO

EXERCISE   YES   NO

HYDRATION

0.5L   1.0L   1.5L   2.0L

Length of Sleep (Hours): (1) (2) (3) (4) (5) (6) (7) (8) (9) (10)

Win of the Day: ....
....

Goals for Tomorrow: ....
....
....

Notes: ....
....
....

Today's Mood: 😠 😟 😧 😐 😊 😃 😄   Day's Rating: ☆☆☆☆☆

Date: ....

FOOD LOG

Breakfast:

YES   NO

SUGAR   YES   NO

EXERCISE   YES   NO

Lunch:

Dinner:

HYDRATION

Snacks:

0.5L   1.0L   1.5L   2.0L

Length of Sleep (Hours): ① ② ③ ④ ⑤ ⑥ ⑦ ⑧ ⑨ ⑩

Win of the Day: ....
....

Goals for Tomorrow: ....
....

Notes: ....
....
....

Today's Mood: 😠 😢 🙁 😐 🙂 😄 😁   Day's Rating: ☆☆☆☆☆

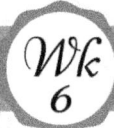
Date: ....

WEIGHT:

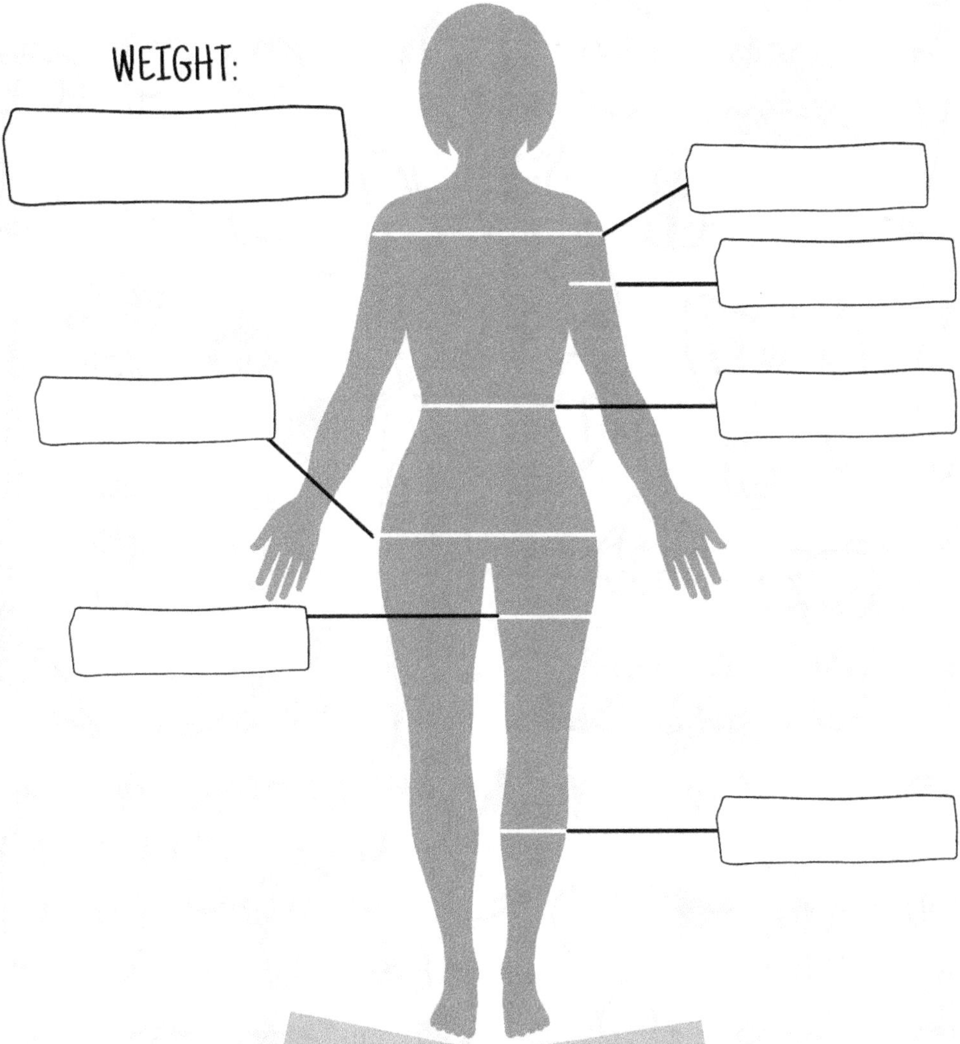

> "A year from now, you will be glad you did not quit today..."

Date: ....

FOOD LOG

Breakfast:

Lunch:

Dinner:

Snacks:

YES   NO

SUGAR   YES   NO

EXERCISE   YES   NO

HYDRATION

0.5L   1.0L   1.5L   2.0L

Length of Sleep (Hours): ① ② ③ ④ ⑤ ⑥ ⑦ ⑧ ⑨ ⑩

Win of the Day: ....
....

Goals for Tomorrow: ....
....

Notes: ....
....
....

Today's Mood: 😠 😞 😟 😐 🙂 😃 😄   Day's Rating: ☆☆☆☆☆

Date: ....

FOOD LOG

Breakfast:

Lunch:

Dinner:

Snacks:

YES   NO

SUGAR   YES   NO

EXERCISE   YES   NO

HYDRATION

0.5L   1.0L   1.5L   2.0L

Length of Sleep (Hours): (1) (2) (3) (4) (5) (6) (7) (8) (9) (10)

Win of the Day: ....
....

Goals for Tomorrow: ....
....

Notes: ....
....
....

Today's Mood: 😠 😢 😕 😐 🙂 😄 😂   Day's Rating: ☆☆☆☆☆☆

Date: ....

FOOD LOG

Breakfast:

YES   NO

Lunch:

SUGAR   YES   NO

EXERCISE   YES   NO

Dinner:

HYDRATION

Snacks:

0.5L   1.0L   1.5L   2.0L

Length of Sleep (Hours): ① ② ③ ④ ⑤ ⑥ ⑦ ⑧ ⑨ ⑩

Win of the Day: ....

....

Goals for Tomorrow: ....

....

Notes: ....

....

Today's Mood: 😠 😟 🙁 😐 🙂 😃 😄   Day's Rating: ☆☆☆☆☆

Date: ....

FOOD LOG

Breakfast:

Lunch:

Dinner:

Snacks:

YES   NO

SUGAR   YES   NO

EXERCISE   YES   NO

HYDRATION

0.5L   1.0L   1.5L   2.0L

Length of Sleep (Hours): ① ② ③ ④ ⑤ ⑥ ⑦ ⑧ ⑨ ⑩

Win of the Day: ....
....

Goals for Tomorrow: ....
....

Notes: ....
....
....

Today's Mood: 😠 😞 😕 😐 🙂 😄 😁   Day's Rating: ☆☆☆☆☆☆

Date: ....

FOOD LOG

Breakfast:

Lunch:

Dinner:

Snacks:

YES   NO

SUGAR   YES   NO

EXERCISE   YES   NO

HYDRATION

0.5L   1.0L   1.5L   2.0L

Length of Sleep (Hours): ① ② ③ ④ ⑤ ⑥ ⑦ ⑧ ⑨ ⑩

Win of the Day: ....

Goals for Tomorrow: ....

Notes: ....

Today's Mood: 😠 🙁 ☹️ 😐 🙂 😄 😁   Day's Rating: ☆☆☆☆☆

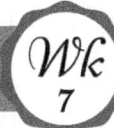
Date: ....

FOOD LOG

Breakfast:

Lunch:

Dinner:

Snacks:

YES   NO

SUGAR   YES   NO

EXERCISE   YES   NO

HYDRATION

0.5L   1.0L   1.5L   2.0L

Length of Sleep (Hours): ① ② ③ ④ ⑤ ⑥ ⑦ ⑧ ⑨ ⑩

Win of the Day: ....
....
....

Goals for Tomorrow: ....
....
....

Notes: ....
....
....

Today's Mood: 😠 😟 😕 😐 🙂 😄 😂   Day's Rating: ☆☆☆☆☆

Daily Health Log

Wk 7

Date:

FOOD LOG

Breakfast:

Lunch:

Dinner:

Snacks:

YES   NO

SUGAR   YES   NO

EXERCISE   YES   NO

HYDRATION

0.5L   1.0L   1.5L   2.0L

Length of Sleep (Hours): 1 2 3 4 5 6 7 8 9 10

Win of the Day:

Goals for Tomorrow:

Notes:

Today's Mood: Day's Rating: ☆☆☆☆☆

Date: ....

WEIGHT:

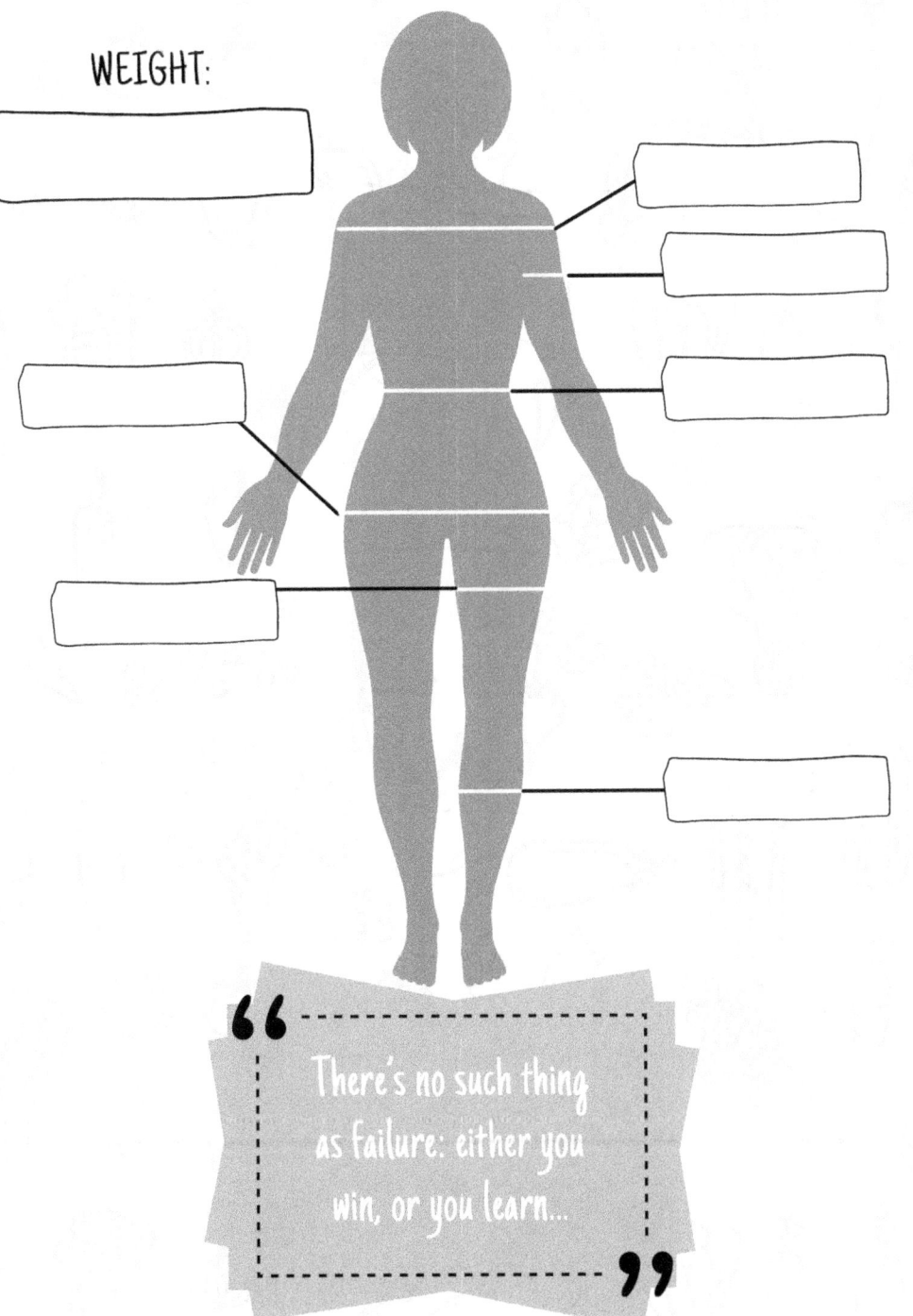

> There's no such thing
> as failure: either you
> win, or you learn...

Date: ....

FOOD LOG

Breakfast:

Lunch:

Dinner:

Snacks:

YES   NO

SUGAR   YES   NO

EXERCISE   YES   NO

HYDRATION

0.5L   1.0L   1.5L   2.0L

Length of Sleep (Hours): (1) (2) (3) (4) (5) (6) (7) (8) (9) (10)

Win of the Day: ....
....

Goals for Tomorrow: ....
....
....

Notes: ....
....
....

Today's Mood: 😠 🙁 ☹️ 😐 🙂 😀 😆   **Day's Rating:** ☆☆☆☆☆

Date: ....

FOOD LOG

Breakfast:

Lunch:

Dinner:

Snacks:

YES   NO

SUGAR   YES   NO

EXERCISE   YES   NO

HYDRATION

0.5L   1.0L   1.5L   2.0L

Length of Sleep (Hours): (1) (2) (3) (4) (5) (6) (7) (8) (9) (10)

Win of the Day: ....
....

Goals for Tomorrow: ....
....

Notes: ....
....
....

Today's Mood: 😠 😟 😣 😐 🙂 😃 😁   Day's Rating: ☆☆☆☆☆

Date: ....

FOOD LOG

Breakfast:

Lunch:

Dinner:

Snacks:

YES   NO

SUGAR   YES   NO

EXERCISE   YES   NO

HYDRATION

0.5L   1.0L   1.5L   2.0L

Length of Sleep (Hours): ① ② ③ ④ ⑤ ⑥ ⑦ ⑧ ⑨ ⑩

Win of the Day: ....

Goals for Tomorrow: ....

Notes: ....

Today's Mood: 😠 😟 🙁 😐 🙂 😃 😄   Day's Rating: ☆☆☆☆☆

Date: ....

FOOD LOG

Breakfast:

Lunch:

Dinner:

Snacks:

🌾 YES NO

SUGAR YES NO

EXERCISE YES NO

HYDRATION

0.5L   1.0L   1.5L   2.0L

Length of Sleep (Hours): ① ② ③ ④ ⑤ ⑥ ⑦ ⑧ ⑨ ⑩

Win of the Day: ....
....

Goals for Tomorrow: ....
....

Notes: ....
....

Today's Mood: 😠 😟 😕 😐 🙂 😄 😆   Day's Rating: ☆☆☆☆☆

Date: ....

FOOD LOG

Breakfast:

Lunch:

Dinner:

Snacks:

YES   NO

SUGAR   YES   NO

EXERCISE   YES   NO

HYDRATION

0.5L   1.0L   1.5L   2.0L

Length of Sleep (Hours): (1) (2) (3) (4) (5) (6) (7) (8) (9) (10)

Win of the Day: ....
....

Goals for Tomorrow: ....
....
....

Notes: ....
....
....

Today's Mood: 😠 😟 🙁 😐 🙂 😄 😁   Day's Rating: ☆☆☆☆☆

Date: ....

FOOD LOG

Breakfast:

 YES   NO

SUGAR   YES   NO

EXERCISE   YES   NO

Lunch:

Dinner:

HYDRATION

Snacks:

0.5L   1.0L   1.5L   2.0L

Length of Sleep (Hours): (1) (2) (3) (4) (5) (6) (7) (8) (9) (10)

Win of the Day: ....
....

Goals for Tomorrow: ....
....
....

Notes: ....
....
....

Today's Mood: 😠 😞 😕 😐 😊 😄 😁   Day's Rating: ☆☆☆☆☆

Date: ....

FOOD LOG

Breakfast:

Lunch:

Dinner:

Snacks:

YES   NO

SUGAR   YES   NO

EXERCISE   YES   NO

HYDRATION

0.5L   1.0L   1.5L   2.0L

Length of Sleep (Hours):   ① ② ③ ④ ⑤ ⑥ ⑦ ⑧ ⑨ ⑩

Win of the Day: ....

....

Goals for Tomorrow: ....

....

Notes: ....

....

....

Today's Mood: 😠 😟 🙁 😐 🙂 😃 😄   Day's Rating: ☆☆☆☆☆

Weekly Weigh-In

Wk 8

Date: ....

WEIGHT:

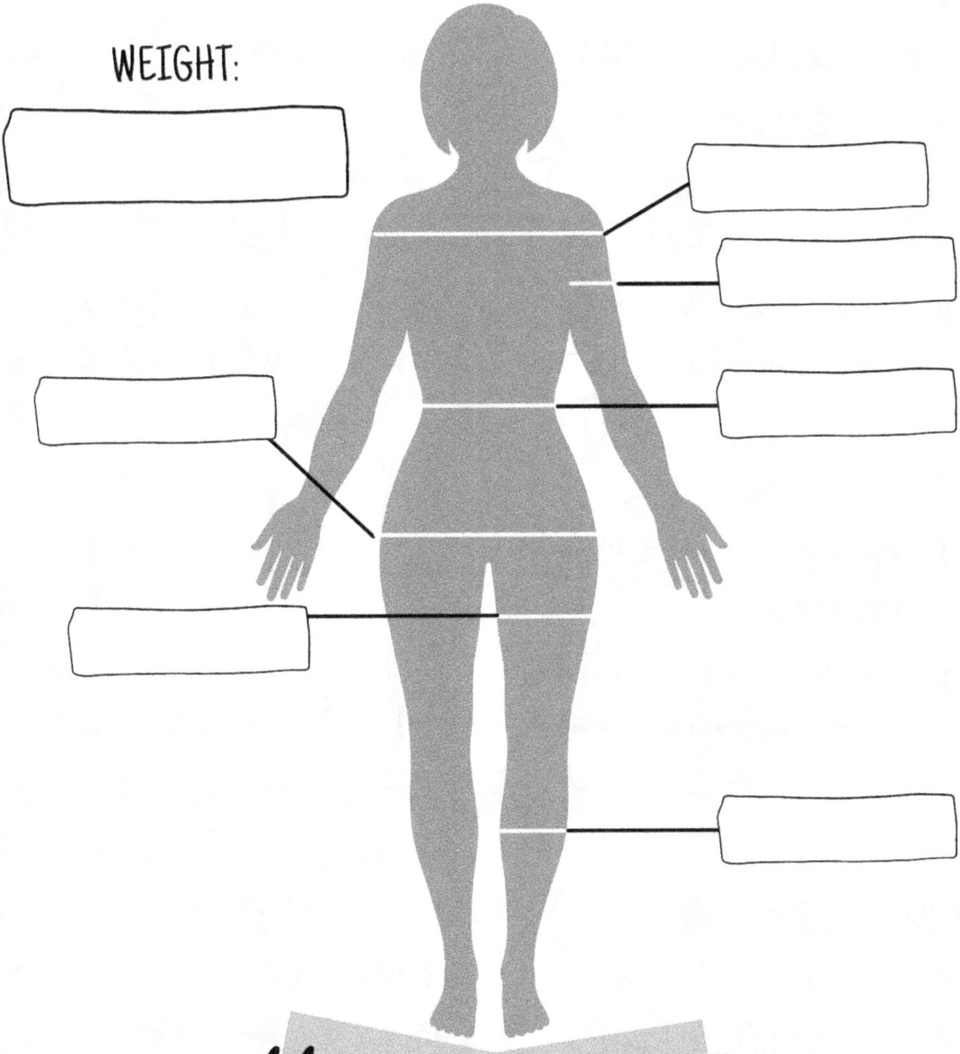

“A little progress each day adds up to big results...”

Wk 9

Date: ....

FOOD LOG

Breakfast:

Lunch:

Dinner:

Snacks:

YES   NO

SUGAR   YES   NO

EXERCISE   YES   NO

HYDRATION

0.5L   1.0L   1.5L   2.0L

Length of Sleep (Hours): ① ② ③ ④ ⑤ ⑥ ⑦ ⑧ ⑨ ⑩

Win of the Day: ....

Goals for Tomorrow: ....

Notes: ....

Today's Mood: 😠 😞 🙁 😐 🙂 😄 😆   Day's Rating: ☆☆☆☆☆

Date: _____

FOOD LOG

Breakfast:

Lunch:

Dinner:

Snacks:

YES NO

SUGAR YES NO

EXERCISE YES NO

HYDRATION

0.5L 1.0L 1.5L 2.0L

Length of Sleep (Hours): (1) (2) (3) (4) (5) (6) (7) (8) (9) (10)

Win of the Day: ....
....

Goals for Tomorrow: ....
....

Notes: ....
....
....

Today's Mood: 😠 😟 😕 😐 🙂 😃 😂   Day's Rating: ☆☆☆☆☆

Date: ....

FOOD LOG

Breakfast:

Lunch:

Dinner:

Snacks:

YES NO

SUGAR YES NO

EXERCISE YES NO

HYDRATION

0.5L 1.0L 1.5L 2.0L

Length of Sleep (Hours): ① ② ③ ④ ⑤ ⑥ ⑦ ⑧ ⑨ ⑩

Win of the Day: ....
....
....

Goals for Tomorrow: ....
....
....

Notes: ....
....
....

Today's Mood: 😠 😟 ☹️ 😐 🙂 😃 😄   Day's Rating: ☆☆☆☆☆

Date: ....

FOOD LOG

Breakfast:

YES   NO

SUGAR   YES   NO

EXERCISE   YES   NO

Lunch:

HYDRATION

Dinner:

Snacks:

0.5L   1.0L   1.5L   2.0L

Length of Sleep (Hours): (1) (2) (3) (4) (5) (6) (7) (8) (9) (10)

Win of the Day: ....
....

Goals for Tomorrow: ....
....
....

Notes: ....
....
....

Today's Mood: 😠 😟 😣 😐 🙂 😃 😄   Day's Rating: ☆☆☆☆☆

Date:

FOOD LOG

Breakfast:

YES   NO

SUGAR   YES   NO

EXERCISE   YES   NO

Lunch:

Dinner:

HYDRATION

Snacks:

0.5L   1.0L   1.5L   2.0L

Length of Sleep (Hours): ① ② ③ ④ ⑤ ⑥ ⑦ ⑧ ⑨ ⑩

Win of the Day:

Goals for Tomorrow:

Notes:

Today's Mood: 😠 😢 🙁 😐 🙂 😄 😁   Day's Rating: ☆☆☆☆☆

Date: ....

FOOD LOG

Breakfast:

YES NO

SUGAR YES NO

EXERCISE YES NO

Lunch:

Dinner:

HYDRATION

Snacks:

0.5L 1.0L 1.5L 2.0L

Length of Sleep (Hours): ① ② ③ ④ ⑤ ⑥ ⑦ ⑧ ⑨ ⑩

Win of the Day: ....

....

Goals for Tomorrow: ....

....

....

Notes: ....

....

....

Today's Mood: 😠 😞 🙁 😐 🙂 😀 😄   Day's Rating: ☆☆☆☆☆☆

Date: ....

FOOD LOG

Breakfast:

Lunch:

Dinner:

Snacks:

YES   NO

SUGAR   YES   NO

EXERCISE   YES   NO

HYDRATION

0.5L   1.0L   1.5L   2.0L

Length of Sleep (Hours): (1) (2) (3) (4) (5) (6) (7) (8) (9) (10)

Win of the Day: ....
....
....

Goals for Tomorrow: ....
....
....

Notes: ....
....
....

Today's Mood: 😠 😢 ☹ 😐 🙂 😀 😄   Day's Rating: ☆☆☆☆☆☆

Weekly Weigh-In

Wk 9

Date: ....

WEIGHT:

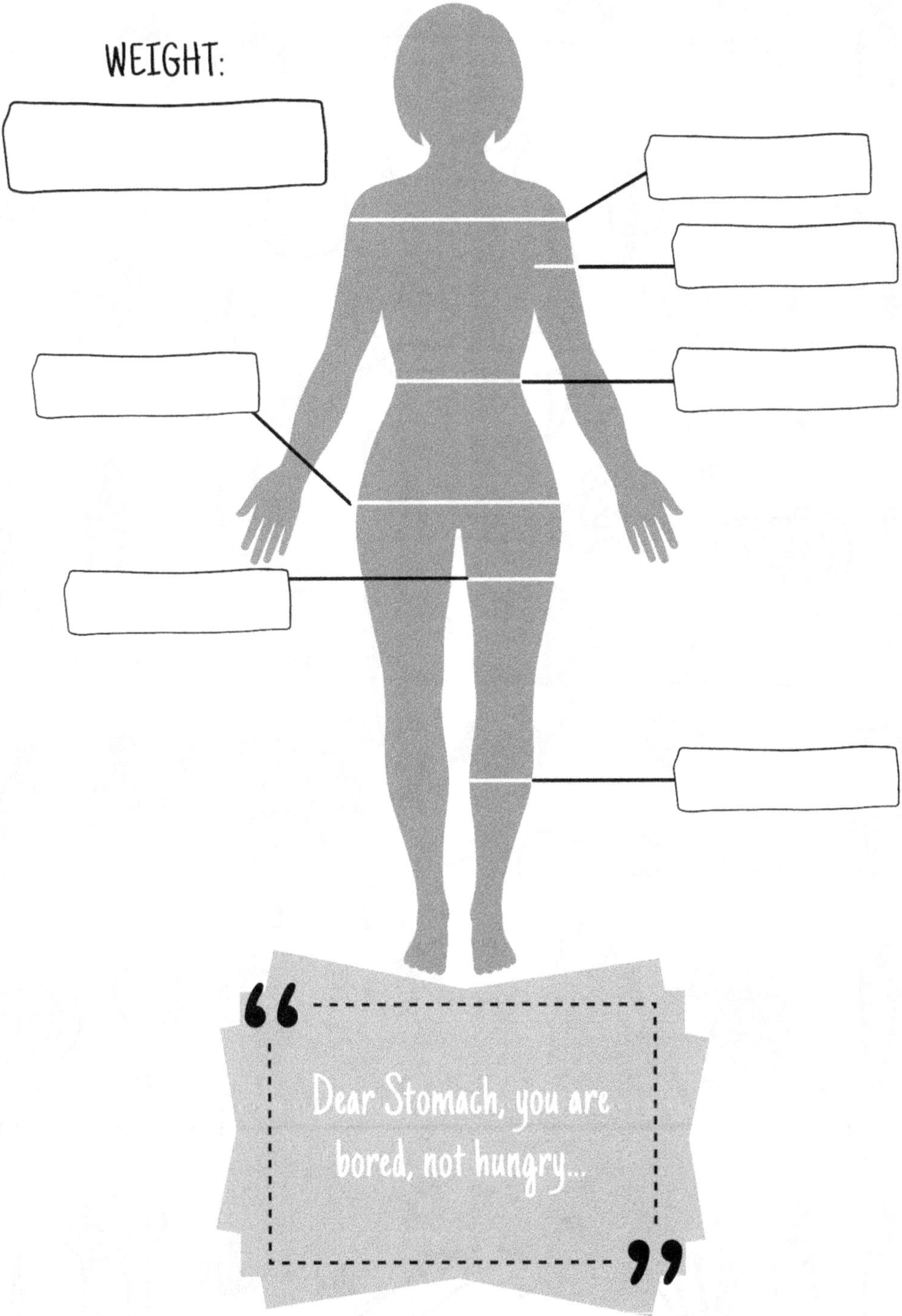

“Dear Stomach, you are bored, not hungry...”

Date: ....

FOOD LOG

Breakfast:

YES   NO

SUGAR   YES   NO

EXERCISE   YES   NO

Lunch:

Dinner:

HYDRATION

Snacks:

0.5L   1.0L   1.5L   2.0L

Length of Sleep (Hours): ① ② ③ ④ ⑤ ⑥ ⑦ ⑧ ⑨ ⑩

Win of the Day: ....
....

Goals for Tomorrow: ....
....

Notes: ....
....
....

Today's Mood: 😠 😟 🙁 😐 🙂 😄 😆   Day's Rating: ☆☆☆☆☆

Daily Health Log

Date: ....

FOOD LOG

Breakfast:

Lunch:

Dinner:

Snacks:

YES   NO

SUGAR   YES   NO

EXERCISE   YES   NO

HYDRATION

0.5L   1.0L   1.5L   2.0L

Length of Sleep (Hours): (1) (2) (3) (4) (5) (6) (7) (8) (9) (10)

Win of the Day: ....
....

Goals for Tomorrow: ....
....

Notes: ....
....
....

Today's Mood: 😠 🙁 😕 😐 🙂 😃 😄   Day's Rating: ☆☆☆☆☆

Date: ....

FOOD LOG

Breakfast:

Lunch:

Dinner:

Snacks:

YES   NO

SUGAR   YES   NO

EXERCISE   YES   NO

HYDRATION

0.5L   1.0L   1.5L   2.0L

Length of Sleep (Hours): (1) (2) (3) (4) (5) (6) (7) (8) (9) (10)

Win of the Day: ....
....

Goals for Tomorrow: ....
....

Notes: ....
....
....

Today's Mood: 😠 😞 ☹️ 😐 🙂 😄 😁   Day's Rating: ☆☆☆☆☆

Date: ....

FOOD LOG

Breakfast:

YES   NO

SUGAR   YES   NO

EXERCISE   YES   NO

Lunch:

Dinner:

HYDRATION

Snacks:

0.5L   1.0L   1.5L   2.0L

Length of Sleep (Hours): ① ② ③ ④ ⑤ ⑥ ⑦ ⑧ ⑨ ⑩

Win of the Day: ....
....

Goals for Tomorrow: ....
....

Notes: ....
....
....

Today's Mood: 😠 😟 🙁 😐 🙂 😄 😁   Day's Rating: ☆☆☆☆☆

Date: ....

FOOD LOG

Breakfast:

YES   NO

Lunch:

SUGAR   YES   NO

EXERCISE   YES   NO

Dinner:

HYDRATION

Snacks:

0.5L   1.0L   1.5L   2.0L

Length of Sleep (Hours): ① ② ③ ④ ⑤ ⑥ ⑦ ⑧ ⑨ ⑩

Win of the Day: ....
....

Goals for Tomorrow: ....
....
....

Notes: ....
....
....

Today's Mood: 😠 😞 😟 😐 🙂 😄 😁   **Day's Rating:** ☆☆☆☆☆

Date: ....

FOOD LOG

Breakfast:

YES NO

Lunch:

SUGAR YES NO

EXERCISE YES NO

Dinner:

HYDRATION

Snacks:

0.5L 1.0L 1.5L 2.0L

Length of Sleep (Hours): ① ② ③ ④ ⑤ ⑥ ⑦ ⑧ ⑨ ⑩

Win of the Day: ....
....

Goals for Tomorrow: ....
....

Notes: ....
....
....

Today's Mood: 😠 ☹️ 😕 😐 🙂 😀 😄   Day's Rating: ☆☆☆☆☆

Daily Health Log

Date:

FOOD LOG

Breakfast:

Lunch:

Dinner:

Snacks:

YES   NO

SUGAR   YES   NO

EXERCISE   YES   NO

HYDRATION

0.5L   1.0L   1.5L   2.0L

Length of Sleep (Hours): ① ② ③ ④ ⑤ ⑥ ⑦ ⑧ ⑨ ⑩

Win of the Day:

Goals for Tomorrow:

Notes:

Today's Mood: 😠 😢 🙁 😐 🙂 😃 😄   Day's Rating: ☆☆☆☆☆

Weekly Weigh-In

Wk 10

Date: ....

WEIGHT:

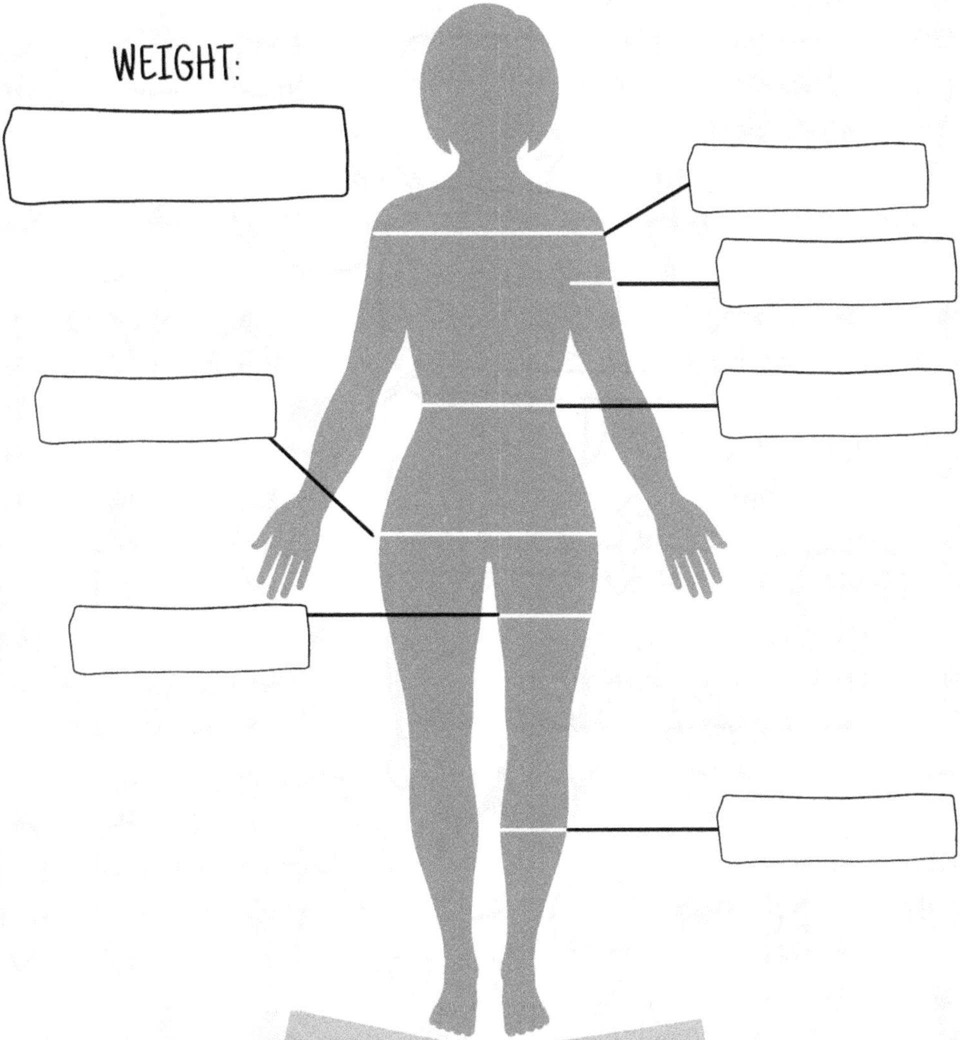

"Turn you head to the left, then to the right.
Repeat this exercise whenever you are offered food...lol"

Date: ....

FOOD LOG

Breakfast:

Lunch:

Dinner:

Snacks:

YES   NO

SUGAR   YES   NO

EXERCISE   YES   NO

HYDRATION

0.5L   1.0L   1.5L   2.0L

Length of Sleep (Hours): ① ② ③ ④ ⑤ ⑥ ⑦ ⑧ ⑨ ⑩

Win of the Day: ....

Goals for Tomorrow: ....

Notes: ....

Today's Mood: 😠 😟 ☹️ 😐 🙂 😄 😁   Day's Rating: ☆☆☆☆☆

Date: ....

FOOD LOG

Breakfast:

Lunch:

Dinner:

Snacks:

YES   NO

SUGAR   YES   NO

EXERCISE   YES   NO

HYDRATION

0.5L   1.0L   1.5L   2.0L

Length of Sleep (Hours): ① ② ③ ④ ⑤ ⑥ ⑦ ⑧ ⑨ ⑩

Win of the Day: ....
....
....

Goals for Tomorrow: ....
....
....

Notes: ....
....
....

Today's Mood: 😠 😟 😕 😐 🙂 😄 😁   Day's Rating: ☆☆☆☆☆☆

Date: ....

FOOD LOG

Breakfast:

Lunch:

Dinner:

Snacks:

YES NO

SUGAR YES NO

EXERCISE YES NO

HYDRATION

0.5L 1.0L 1.5L 2.0L

Length of Sleep (Hours): (1) (2) (3) (4) (5) (6) (7) (8) (9) (10)

Win of the Day: ....

Goals for Tomorrow: ....

Notes: ....

Today's Mood: 😠 😣 🙁 😐 🙂 😄 😆   Day's Rating: ☆☆☆☆☆

Daily Health Log

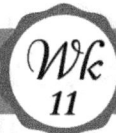

Wk 11

Date: ....

FOOD LOG

Breakfast:

Lunch:

Dinner:

Snacks:

YES   NO

SUGAR   YES   NO

EXERCISE   YES   NO

HYDRATION

0.5L   1.0L   1.5L   2.0L

Length of Sleep (Hours): (1) (2) (3) (4) (5) (6) (7) (8) (9) (10)

Win of the Day: ....
....

Goals for Tomorrow: ....
....

Notes: ....
....
....

Today's Mood: 😠 😞 😕 😐 🙂 😄 😂   Day's Rating: ☆☆☆☆☆

Date: ....

FOOD LOG

Breakfast:

Lunch:

Dinner:

Snacks:

YES NO

SUGAR YES NO

EXERCISE YES NO

HYDRATION

0.5L   1.0L   1.5L   2.0L

Length of Sleep (Hours): (1) (2) (3) (4) (5) (6) (7) (8) (9) (10)

Win of the Day: ....

Goals for Tomorrow: ....

Notes: ....

Today's Mood: 😠 😟 😞 😐 🙂 😄 😆   **Day's Rating:** ☆☆☆☆☆

Date: ....

FOOD LOG

Breakfast:

Lunch:

Dinner:

Snacks:

YES   NO

SUGAR   YES   NO

EXERCISE   YES   NO

HYDRATION

0.5L   1.0L   1.5L   2.0L

Length of Sleep (Hours): ① ② ③ ④ ⑤ ⑥ ⑦ ⑧ ⑨ ⑩

Win of the Day: ....

....

Goals for Tomorrow: ....

....

Notes: ....

....

Today's Mood: 😠 😟 🙁 😐 🙂 😃 😄   Day's Rating: ☆☆☆☆☆☆

Date: ....

FOOD LOG

Breakfast:

YES   NO

Lunch:

SUGAR   YES   NO

EXERCISE   YES   NO

Dinner:

HYDRATION

Snacks:

0.5L   1.0L   1.5L   2.0L

Length of Sleep (Hours): ① ② ③ ④ ⑤ ⑥ ⑦ ⑧ ⑨ ⑩

Win of the Day: ....
....

Goals for Tomorrow: ....
....

Notes: ....
....
....

Today's Mood: 😠 😟 🙁 😐 🙂 😃 😄   Day's Rating: ☆☆☆☆☆

Weekly Weigh-In

Wk 11

Date: ....

WEIGHT:

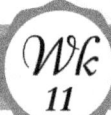

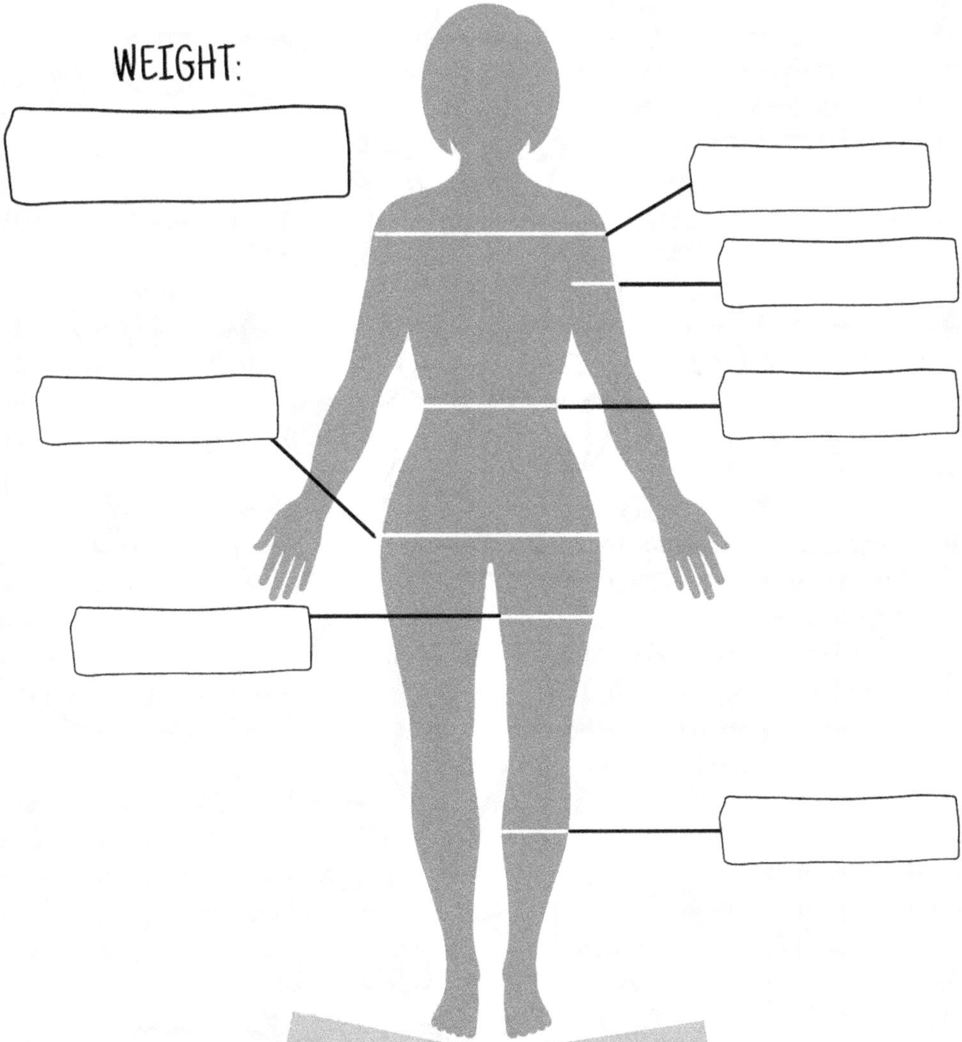

"Whatever the problem is, the answer is not in the fridge..."

FOOD LOG

Date: ....

Breakfast:

Lunch:

Dinner:

Snacks:

YES   NO

SUGAR   YES   NO

EXERCISE   YES   NO

HYDRATION

0.5L   1.0L   1.5L   2.0L

Length of Sleep (Hours): ① ② ③ ④ ⑤ ⑥ ⑦ ⑧ ⑨ ⑩

Win of the Day: ....

Goals for Tomorrow: ....

Notes: ....

Today's Mood: 😠 😢 🙁 😐 🙂 😀 😆   Day's Rating: ☆☆☆☆☆☆

Date: ....

FOOD LOG

Breakfast:

Lunch:

Dinner:

Snacks:

YES   NO

SUGAR   YES   NO

EXERCISE   YES   NO

HYDRATION

0.5L   1.0L   1.5L   2.0L

Length of Sleep (Hours): ① ② ③ ④ ⑤ ⑥ ⑦ ⑧ ⑨ ⑩

Win of the Day: ....
....

Goals for Tomorrow: ....
....

Notes: ....
....
....

Today's Mood: 😠 😟 🙁 😐 🙂 😃 😄   Day's Rating: ☆☆☆☆☆☆

Date: ....

FOOD LOG

Breakfast:

YES   NO

Lunch:

SUGAR   YES   NO

EXERCISE   YES   NO

Dinner:

HYDRATION

Snacks:

0.5L   1.0L   1.5L   2.0L

Length of Sleep (Hours): ① ② ③ ④ ⑤ ⑥ ⑦ ⑧ ⑨ ⑩

Win of the Day: ....
....

Goals for Tomorrow: ....
....
....

Notes: ....
....
....

Today's Mood: 😠 😢 🙁 😐 🙂 😃 😄   Day's Rating: ☆☆☆☆☆

Date: ....

FOOD LOG

Breakfast:

YES   NO

SUGAR   YES   NO

EXERCISE   YES   NO

Lunch:

Dinner:

HYDRATION

Snacks:

0.5L   1.0L   1.5L   2.0L

Length of Sleep (Hours): (1) (2) (3) (4) (5) (6) (7) (8) (9) (10)

Win of the Day: ....
....

Goals for Tomorrow: ....
....

Notes: ....
....
....

Today's Mood: 😠 😟 🙁 😐 🙂 😄 😁   Day's Rating: ☆☆☆☆☆

Date: ....

FOOD LOG

Breakfast:

YES   NO

Lunch:

SUGAR   YES   NO

EXERCISE   YES   NO

Dinner:

HYDRATION

Snacks:

0.5L   1.0L   1.5L   2.0L

Length of Sleep (Hours): (1) (2) (3) (4) (5) (6) (7) (8) (9) (10)

Win of the Day: ....

Goals for Tomorrow: ....

Notes: ....

Today's Mood: 😠 😟 🙁 😐 🙂 😄   **Day's Rating:** ☆☆☆☆☆

FOOD LOG

Date: ....

Breakfast:

Lunch:

Dinner:

Snacks:

YES   NO

SUGAR   YES   NO

EXERCISE   YES   NO

HYDRATION

0.5L   1.0L   1.5L   2.0L

Length of Sleep (Hours): (1) (2) (3) (4) (5) (6) (7) (8) (9) (10)

Win of the Day: ....
....

Goals for Tomorrow: ....
....

Notes: ....
....
....

Today's Mood: 😠 😟 🙁 😐 🙂 😃 😄   Day's Rating: ☆☆☆☆☆☆

Date: ....

FOOD LOG

Breakfast:

Lunch:

Dinner:

Snacks:

YES NO

SUGAR YES NO

EXERCISE YES NO

HYDRATION

0.5L 1.0L 1.5L 2.0L

Length of Sleep (Hours): ① ② ③ ④ ⑤ ⑥ ⑦ ⑧ ⑨ ⑩

Win of the Day: ....
....

Goals for Tomorrow: ....
....

Notes: ....
....
....

Today's Mood: 😠 😟 🙁 😐 🙂 😄 😁   Day's Rating: ☆☆☆☆☆☆

Date: ....

WEIGHT:

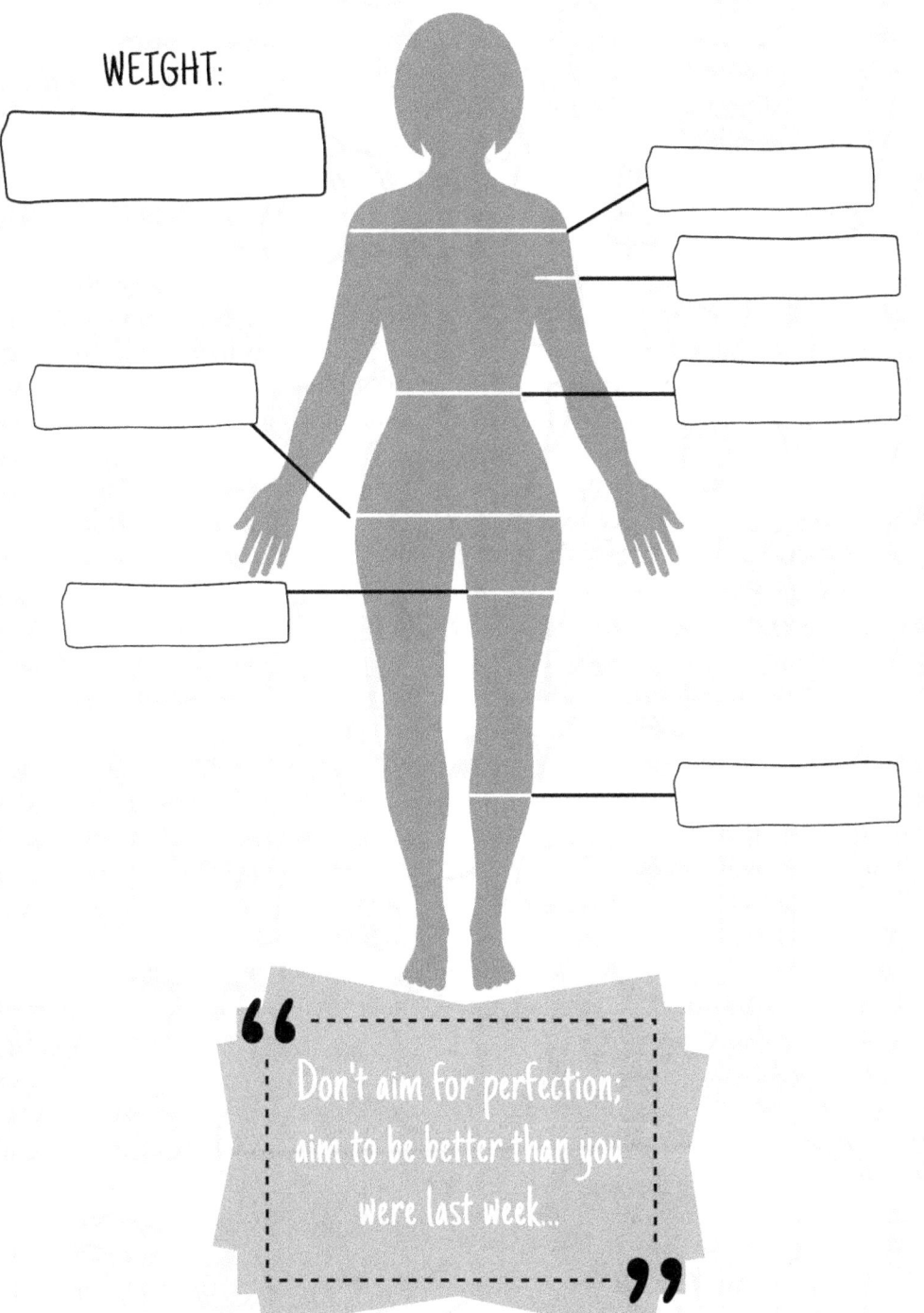

> Don't aim for perfection;
> aim to be better than you
> were last week...

www.ingramcontent.com/pod-product-compliance
Lightning Source LLC
Chambersburg PA
CBHW070428290526
45791CB00005B/1890